Grandad's Blood Sugar Logbook

Dubreck World Publishing

Copyright

'Grandad's Blood Sugar Logbook'

First published in July 2021 by Dubreck World Publishing
Printed and bound by Lulu Press
Distributed by Lulu Press

ISBN-13: 978-1-105-71073-5

First Edition

DUBRECK WORLD PUBLISHING

For Grandad

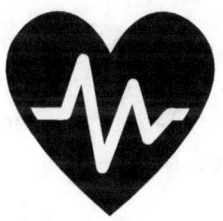

Blood Sugar Monitoring

Regularly record your levels in this logbook and take it with you to your next doctor or nurse appointment. This will help them see your overall progress and consider if any adjustment to your treatment may be necessary.

Record your blood sugar levels as often as you are advised to by a qualified medical practitioner.

Understanding Your Blood Sugar Levels

Blood sugar levels are also often referred to as blood glucose levels. By monitoring your levels, you are better able to manage your diabetes to reduce both acute and more longer term complications.

Glucose is a sugar found in many drinks and foods, and the levels you are monitoring indicates how much glucose is in your blood at that moment of measurement. The level will change throughout the day, depending on factors such as what you have eaten or drank, your level of activity, your current state of health etc. In people with diabetes, the high and low blood sugar levels reached can be much greater and more frequent than in people without diabetes.

As a person with diabetes, regularly checking your blood sugar levels will allow you to recognise when they become too low (hypoglycaemia) or too high (hyperglycaemia), and will allow you to take action, as advised by your medical practitioner, before the situation becomes serious. It may also help you to understand patterns in your blood sugar levels, which will help you manage your diabetes, stay healthy, and avoid future complications.

What Should Your Blood Sugar Levels Be?

Usually, the best time to check your blood sugar levels is before mealtimes. Check them as directed by your medical practitioner.

Under 4 mmol/l	**Too Low**
4 – 7 mmol/l	**Healthy Target**
Over 7 mmol/l	**Too High**

These are blood sugar level targets for adults with type 1 and type 2 diabetes. Your individual targets may differ.

Personal Details

Personal

Name_____

Address_____

_____

_____

Tel_____

Email_____

D.O.B._____

Medical

Doctor's Name_____

Doctor's Surgery_____

Doctor's Tel_____

Emergency Contact

First Contact:

Name_____

Phone_____

Second Contact:

Name_____

Phone_____

Blood Sugar Log

Example

Week: 26th July 2021

Monday

Time	Before	After	Notes
Breakfast	4.6		Feeling well
Lunch			
Dinner			
Bedtime			
Snacks			

1. Week:

Monday

Time	Before	After	Notes
Breakfast			
Lunch			
Dinner			
Bedtime			
Snacks			

Tuesday

Time	Before	After	Notes
Breakfast			
Lunch			
Dinner			
Bedtime			
Snacks			

Wednesday

Time	Before	After	Notes
Breakfast			
Lunch			
Dinner			
Bedtime			
Snacks			

Thursday

Time	Before	After	Notes
Breakfast			
Lunch			
Dinner			
Bedtime			
Snacks			

Friday

Time	Before	After	Notes
Breakfast			
Lunch			
Dinner			
Bedtime			
Snacks			

Saturday

Time	Before	After	Notes
Breakfast			
Lunch			
Dinner			
Bedtime			
Snacks			

Sunday

Time	Before	After	Notes
Breakfast			
Lunch			
Dinner			
Bedtime			
Snacks			

Notes

2. Week:

Monday

Time	Before	After	Notes
Breakfast			
Lunch			
Dinner			
Bedtime			
Snacks			

Tuesday

Time	Before	After	Notes
Breakfast			
Lunch			
Dinner			
Bedtime			
Snacks			

Wednesday

Time	Before	After	Notes
Breakfast			
Lunch			
Dinner			
Bedtime			
Snacks			

Thursday

Time	Before	After	Notes
Breakfast			
Lunch			
Dinner			
Bedtime			
Snacks			

Friday

Time	Before	After	Notes
Breakfast			
Lunch			
Dinner			
Bedtime			
Snacks			

Saturday

Time	Before	After	Notes
Breakfast			
Lunch			
Dinner			
Bedtime			
Snacks			

Sunday

Time	Before	After	Notes
Breakfast			
Lunch			
Dinner			
Bedtime			
Snacks			

Notes

3. Week:

Monday

Time	Before	After	Notes
Breakfast			
Lunch			
Dinner			
Bedtime			
Snacks			

Tuesday

Time	Before	After	Notes
Breakfast			
Lunch			
Dinner			
Bedtime			
Snacks			

Wednesday

Time	Before	After	Notes
Breakfast			
Lunch			
Dinner			
Bedtime			
Snacks			

Thursday

Time	Before	After	Notes
Breakfast			
Lunch			
Dinner			
Bedtime			
Snacks			

Friday

Time	Before	After	Notes
Breakfast			
Lunch			
Dinner			
Bedtime			
Snacks			

Saturday

Time	Before	After	Notes
Breakfast			
Lunch			
Dinner			
Bedtime			
Snacks			

Sunday

Time	Before	After	Notes
Breakfast			
Lunch			
Dinner			
Bedtime			
Snacks			

Notes

4. Week:

Monday

Time	Before	After	Notes
Breakfast			
Lunch			
Dinner			
Bedtime			
Snacks			

Tuesday

Time	Before	After	Notes
Breakfast			
Lunch			
Dinner			
Bedtime			
Snacks			

Wednesday

Time	Before	After	Notes
Breakfast			
Lunch			
Dinner			
Bedtime			
Snacks			

Thursday

Time	Before	After	Notes
Breakfast			
Lunch			
Dinner			
Bedtime			
Snacks			

Friday

Time	Before	After	Notes
Breakfast			
Lunch			
Dinner			
Bedtime			
Snacks			

Saturday

Time	Before	After	Notes
Breakfast			
Lunch			
Dinner			
Bedtime			
Snacks			

Sunday

Time	Before	After	Notes
Breakfast			
Lunch			
Dinner			
Bedtime			
Snacks			

Notes

5. Week:

Monday

Time	Before	After	Notes
Breakfast			
Lunch			
Dinner			
Bedtime			
Snacks			

Tuesday

Time	Before	After	Notes
Breakfast			
Lunch			
Dinner			
Bedtime			
Snacks			

Wednesday

Time	Before	After	Notes
Breakfast			
Lunch			
Dinner			
Bedtime			
Snacks			

Thursday

Time	Before	After	Notes
Breakfast			
Lunch			
Dinner			
Bedtime			
Snacks			

Friday

Time	Before	After	Notes
Breakfast			
Lunch			
Dinner			
Bedtime			
Snacks			

Saturday

Time	Before	After	Notes
Breakfast			
Lunch			
Dinner			
Bedtime			
Snacks			

Sunday

Time	Before	After	Notes
Breakfast			
Lunch			
Dinner			
Bedtime			
Snacks			

Notes

6. Week:

Monday

Time	Before	After	Notes
Breakfast			
Lunch			
Dinner			
Bedtime			
Snacks			

Tuesday

Time	Before	After	Notes
Breakfast			
Lunch			
Dinner			
Bedtime			
Snacks			

Wednesday

Time	Before	After	Notes
Breakfast			
Lunch			
Dinner			
Bedtime			
Snacks			

Thursday

Time	Before	After	Notes
Breakfast			
Lunch			
Dinner			
Bedtime			
Snacks			

Friday

Time	Before	After	Notes
Breakfast			
Lunch			
Dinner			
Bedtime			
Snacks			

Saturday

Time	Before	After	Notes
Breakfast			
Lunch			
Dinner			
Bedtime			
Snacks			

Sunday

Time	Before	After	Notes
Breakfast			
Lunch			
Dinner			
Bedtime			
Snacks			

Notes

7. Week:

Monday

Time	Before	After	Notes
Breakfast			
Lunch			
Dinner			
Bedtime			
Snacks			

Tuesday

Time	Before	After	Notes
Breakfast			
Lunch			
Dinner			
Bedtime			
Snacks			

Wednesday

Time	Before	After	Notes
Breakfast			
Lunch			
Dinner			
Bedtime			
Snacks			

Thursday

Time	Before	After	Notes
Breakfast			
Lunch			
Dinner			
Bedtime			
Snacks			

Friday

Time	Before	After	Notes
Breakfast			
Lunch			
Dinner			
Bedtime			
Snacks			

Saturday

Time	Before	After	Notes
Breakfast			
Lunch			
Dinner			
Bedtime			
Snacks			

Sunday

Time	Before	After	Notes
Breakfast			
Lunch			
Dinner			
Bedtime			
Snacks			

Notes

8. Week:

Monday

Time	Before	After	Notes
Breakfast			
Lunch			
Dinner			
Bedtime			
Snacks			

Tuesday

Time	Before	After	Notes
Breakfast			
Lunch			
Dinner			
Bedtime			
Snacks			

Wednesday

Time	Before	After	Notes
Breakfast			
Lunch			
Dinner			
Bedtime			
Snacks			

Thursday

Time	Before	After	Notes
Breakfast			
Lunch			
Dinner			
Bedtime			
Snacks			

Friday

Time	Before	After	Notes
Breakfast			
Lunch			
Dinner			
Bedtime			
Snacks			

Saturday

Time	Before	After	Notes
Breakfast			
Lunch			
Dinner			
Bedtime			
Snacks			

Sunday

Time	Before	After	Notes
Breakfast			
Lunch			
Dinner			
Bedtime			
Snacks			

Notes

9. Week:

Monday

Time	Before	After	Notes
Breakfast			
Lunch			
Dinner			
Bedtime			
Snacks			

Tuesday

Time	Before	After	Notes
Breakfast			
Lunch			
Dinner			
Bedtime			
Snacks			

Wednesday

Time	Before	After	Notes
Breakfast			
Lunch			
Dinner			
Bedtime			
Snacks			

Thursday

Time	Before	After	Notes
Breakfast			
Lunch			
Dinner			
Bedtime			
Snacks			

Friday

Time	Before	After	Notes
Breakfast			
Lunch			
Dinner			
Bedtime			
Snacks			

Saturday

Time	Before	After	Notes
Breakfast			
Lunch			
Dinner			
Bedtime			
Snacks			

Sunday

Time	Before	After	Notes
Breakfast			
Lunch			
Dinner			
Bedtime			
Snacks			

Notes

10. Week:

Monday

Time	Before	After	Notes
Breakfast			
Lunch			
Dinner			
Bedtime			
Snacks			

Tuesday

Time	Before	After	Notes
Breakfast			
Lunch			
Dinner			
Bedtime			
Snacks			

Wednesday

Time	Before	After	Notes
Breakfast			
Lunch			
Dinner			
Bedtime			
Snacks			

Thursday

Time	Before	After	Notes
Breakfast			
Lunch			
Dinner			
Bedtime			
Snacks			

Friday

Time	Before	After	Notes
Breakfast			
Lunch			
Dinner			
Bedtime			
Snacks			

Saturday

Time	Before	After	Notes
Breakfast			
Lunch			
Dinner			
Bedtime			
Snacks			

Sunday

Time	Before	After	Notes
Breakfast			
Lunch			
Dinner			
Bedtime			
Snacks			

Notes

11.   Week:

Monday

Time	Before	After	Notes
Breakfast			
Lunch			
Dinner			
Bedtime			
Snacks			

Tuesday

Time	Before	After	Notes
Breakfast			
Lunch			
Dinner			
Bedtime			
Snacks			

Wednesday

Time	Before	After	Notes
Breakfast			
Lunch			
Dinner			
Bedtime			
Snacks			

Thursday

Time	Before	After	Notes
Breakfast			
Lunch			
Dinner			
Bedtime			
Snacks			

Friday

Time	Before	After	Notes
Breakfast			
Lunch			
Dinner			
Bedtime			
Snacks			

Saturday

Time	Before	After	Notes
Breakfast			
Lunch			
Dinner			
Bedtime			
Snacks			

Sunday

Time	Before	After	Notes
Breakfast			
Lunch			
Dinner			
Bedtime			
Snacks			

Notes

12.   Week:

Monday

Time	Before	After	Notes
Breakfast			
Lunch			
Dinner			
Bedtime			
Snacks			

Tuesday

Time	Before	After	Notes
Breakfast			
Lunch			
Dinner			
Bedtime			
Snacks			

Wednesday

Time	Before	After	Notes
Breakfast			
Lunch			
Dinner			
Bedtime			
Snacks			

Thursday

Time	Before	After	Notes
Breakfast			
Lunch			
Dinner			
Bedtime			
Snacks			

Friday

Time	Before	After	Notes
Breakfast			
Lunch			
Dinner			
Bedtime			
Snacks			

Saturday

Time	Before	After	Notes
Breakfast			
Lunch			
Dinner			
Bedtime			
Snacks			

Sunday

Time	Before	After	Notes
Breakfast			
Lunch			
Dinner			
Bedtime			
Snacks			

Notes

13.   Week:

Monday

Time	Before	After	Notes
Breakfast			
Lunch			
Dinner			
Bedtime			
Snacks			

Tuesday

Time	Before	After	Notes
Breakfast			
Lunch			
Dinner			
Bedtime			
Snacks			

Wednesday

Time	Before	After	Notes
Breakfast			
Lunch			
Dinner			
Bedtime			
Snacks			

Thursday

Time	Before	After	Notes
Breakfast			
Lunch			
Dinner			
Bedtime			
Snacks			

Friday

Time	Before	After	Notes
Breakfast			
Lunch			
Dinner			
Bedtime			
Snacks			

Saturday

Time	Before	After	Notes
Breakfast			
Lunch			
Dinner			
Bedtime			
Snacks			

Sunday

Time	Before	After	Notes
Breakfast			
Lunch			
Dinner			
Bedtime			
Snacks			

Notes

14.   Week:

Monday

Time	Before	After	Notes
Breakfast			
Lunch			
Dinner			
Bedtime			
Snacks			

Tuesday

Time	Before	After	Notes
Breakfast			
Lunch			
Dinner			
Bedtime			
Snacks			

Wednesday

Time	Before	After	Notes
Breakfast			
Lunch			
Dinner			
Bedtime			
Snacks			

Thursday

Time	Before	After	Notes
Breakfast			
Lunch			
Dinner			
Bedtime			
Snacks			

Friday

Time	Before	After	Notes
Breakfast			
Lunch			
Dinner			
Bedtime			
Snacks			

Saturday

Time	Before	After	Notes
Breakfast			
Lunch			
Dinner			
Bedtime			
Snacks			

Sunday

Time	Before	After	Notes
Breakfast			
Lunch			
Dinner			
Bedtime			
Snacks			

Notes

15.   Week:

Monday

Time	Before	After	Notes
Breakfast			
Lunch			
Dinner			
Bedtime			
Snacks			

Tuesday

Time	Before	After	Notes
Breakfast			
Lunch			
Dinner			
Bedtime			
Snacks			

Wednesday

Time	Before	After	Notes
Breakfast			
Lunch			
Dinner			
Bedtime			
Snacks			

Thursday

Time	Before	After	Notes
Breakfast			
Lunch			
Dinner			
Bedtime			
Snacks			

Friday

Time	Before	After	Notes
Breakfast			
Lunch			
Dinner			
Bedtime			
Snacks			

Saturday

Time	Before	After	Notes
Breakfast			
Lunch			
Dinner			
Bedtime			
Snacks			

Sunday

Time	Before	After	Notes
Breakfast			
Lunch			
Dinner			
Bedtime			
Snacks			

Notes

16.   Week:

Monday

Time	Before	After	Notes
Breakfast			
Lunch			
Dinner			
Bedtime			
Snacks			

Tuesday

Time	Before	After	Notes
Breakfast			
Lunch			
Dinner			
Bedtime			
Snacks			

Wednesday

Time	Before	After	Notes
Breakfast			
Lunch			
Dinner			
Bedtime			
Snacks			

Thursday

Time	Before	After	Notes
Breakfast			
Lunch			
Dinner			
Bedtime			
Snacks			

Friday

Time	Before	After	Notes
Breakfast			
Lunch			
Dinner			
Bedtime			
Snacks			

Saturday

Time	Before	After	Notes
Breakfast			
Lunch			
Dinner			
Bedtime			
Snacks			

Sunday

Time	Before	After	Notes
Breakfast			
Lunch			
Dinner			
Bedtime			
Snacks			

Notes

17.   Week:

Monday

Time	Before	After	Notes
Breakfast			
Lunch			
Dinner			
Bedtime			
Snacks			

Tuesday

Time	Before	After	Notes
Breakfast			
Lunch			
Dinner			
Bedtime			
Snacks			

Wednesday

Time	Before	After	Notes
Breakfast			
Lunch			
Dinner			
Bedtime			
Snacks			

Thursday

Time	Before	After	Notes
Breakfast			
Lunch			
Dinner			
Bedtime			
Snacks			

Friday

Time	Before	After	Notes
Breakfast			
Lunch			
Dinner			
Bedtime			
Snacks			

Saturday

Time	Before	After	Notes
Breakfast			
Lunch			
Dinner			
Bedtime			
Snacks			

Sunday

Time	Before	After	Notes
Breakfast			
Lunch			
Dinner			
Bedtime			
Snacks			

Notes

18.   Week:

Monday

Time	Before	After	Notes
Breakfast			
Lunch			
Dinner			
Bedtime			
Snacks			

Tuesday

Time	Before	After	Notes
Breakfast			
Lunch			
Dinner			
Bedtime			
Snacks			

Wednesday

Time	Before	After	Notes
Breakfast			
Lunch			
Dinner			
Bedtime			
Snacks			

Thursday

Time	Before	After	Notes
Breakfast			
Lunch			
Dinner			
Bedtime			
Snacks			

Friday

Time	Before	After	Notes
Breakfast			
Lunch			
Dinner			
Bedtime			
Snacks			

Saturday

Time	Before	After	Notes
Breakfast			
Lunch			
Dinner			
Bedtime			
Snacks			

Sunday

Time	Before	After	Notes
Breakfast			
Lunch			
Dinner			
Bedtime			
Snacks			

Notes

19.   Week:

Monday

Time	Before	After	Notes
Breakfast			
Lunch			
Dinner			
Bedtime			
Snacks			

Tuesday

Time	Before	After	Notes
Breakfast			
Lunch			
Dinner			
Bedtime			
Snacks			

Wednesday

Time	Before	After	Notes
Breakfast			
Lunch			
Dinner			
Bedtime			
Snacks			

Thursday

Time	Before	After	Notes
Breakfast			
Lunch			
Dinner			
Bedtime			
Snacks			

Friday

Time	Before	After	Notes
Breakfast			
Lunch			
Dinner			
Bedtime			
Snacks			

Saturday

Time	Before	After	Notes
Breakfast			
Lunch			
Dinner			
Bedtime			
Snacks			

Sunday

Time	Before	After	Notes
Breakfast			
Lunch			
Dinner			
Bedtime			
Snacks			

Notes

20.   Week:

Monday

Time	Before	After	Notes
Breakfast			
Lunch			
Dinner			
Bedtime			
Snacks			

Tuesday

Time	Before	After	Notes
Breakfast			
Lunch			
Dinner			
Bedtime			
Snacks			

Wednesday

Time	Before	After	Notes
Breakfast			
Lunch			
Dinner			
Bedtime			
Snacks			

Thursday

Time	Before	After	Notes
Breakfast			
Lunch			
Dinner			
Bedtime			
Snacks			

Friday

Time	Before	After	Notes
Breakfast			
Lunch			
Dinner			
Bedtime			
Snacks			

Saturday

Time	Before	After	Notes
Breakfast			
Lunch			
Dinner			
Bedtime			
Snacks			

Sunday

Time	Before	After	Notes
Breakfast			
Lunch			
Dinner			
Bedtime			
Snacks			

Notes

21.   Week:

Monday

Time	Before	After	Notes
Breakfast			
Lunch			
Dinner			
Bedtime			
Snacks			

Tuesday

Time	Before	After	Notes
Breakfast			
Lunch			
Dinner			
Bedtime			
Snacks			

Wednesday

Time	Before	After	Notes
Breakfast			
Lunch			
Dinner			
Bedtime			
Snacks			

Thursday

Time	Before	After	Notes
Breakfast			
Lunch			
Dinner			
Bedtime			
Snacks			

Friday

Time	Before	After	Notes
Breakfast			
Lunch			
Dinner			
Bedtime			
Snacks			

Saturday

Time	Before	After	Notes
Breakfast			
Lunch			
Dinner			
Bedtime			
Snacks			

Sunday

Time	Before	After	Notes
Breakfast			
Lunch			
Dinner			
Bedtime			
Snacks			

Notes

22.   Week:

Monday

Time	Before	After	Notes
Breakfast			
Lunch			
Dinner			
Bedtime			
Snacks			

Tuesday

Time	Before	After	Notes
Breakfast			
Lunch			
Dinner			
Bedtime			
Snacks			

Wednesday

Time	Before	After	Notes
Breakfast			
Lunch			
Dinner			
Bedtime			
Snacks			

Thursday

Time	Before	After	Notes
Breakfast			
Lunch			
Dinner			
Bedtime			
Snacks			

Friday

Time	Before	After	Notes
Breakfast			
Lunch			
Dinner			
Bedtime			
Snacks			

Saturday

Time	Before	After	Notes
Breakfast			
Lunch			
Dinner			
Bedtime			
Snacks			

Sunday

Time	Before	After	Notes
Breakfast			
Lunch			
Dinner			
Bedtime			
Snacks			

Notes

23.   Week:

Monday

Time	Before	After	Notes
Breakfast			
Lunch			
Dinner			
Bedtime			
Snacks			

Tuesday

Time	Before	After	Notes
Breakfast			
Lunch			
Dinner			
Bedtime			
Snacks			

Wednesday

Time	Before	After	Notes
Breakfast			
Lunch			
Dinner			
Bedtime			
Snacks			

Thursday

Time	Before	After	Notes
Breakfast			
Lunch			
Dinner			
Bedtime			
Snacks			

Friday

Time	Before	After	Notes
Breakfast			
Lunch			
Dinner			
Bedtime			
Snacks			

Saturday

Time	Before	After	Notes
Breakfast			
Lunch			
Dinner			
Bedtime			
Snacks			

Sunday

Time	Before	After	Notes
Breakfast			
Lunch			
Dinner			
Bedtime			
Snacks			

Notes

24. Week:

Monday

Time	Before	After	Notes
Breakfast			
Lunch			
Dinner			
Bedtime			
Snacks			

Tuesday

Time	Before	After	Notes
Breakfast			
Lunch			
Dinner			
Bedtime			
Snacks			

Wednesday

Time	Before	After	Notes
Breakfast			
Lunch			
Dinner			
Bedtime			
Snacks			

Thursday

Time	Before	After	Notes
Breakfast			
Lunch			
Dinner			
Bedtime			
Snacks			

Friday

Time	Before	After	Notes
Breakfast			
Lunch			
Dinner			
Bedtime			
Snacks			

Saturday

Time	Before	After	Notes
Breakfast			
Lunch			
Dinner			
Bedtime			
Snacks			

Sunday

Time	Before	After	Notes
Breakfast			
Lunch			
Dinner			
Bedtime			
Snacks			

Notes

25.   Week:

Monday

Time	Before	After	Notes
Breakfast			
Lunch			
Dinner			
Bedtime			
Snacks			

Tuesday

Time	Before	After	Notes
Breakfast			
Lunch			
Dinner			
Bedtime			
Snacks			

Wednesday

Time	Before	After	Notes
Breakfast			
Lunch			
Dinner			
Bedtime			
Snacks			

Thursday

Time	Before	After	Notes
Breakfast			
Lunch			
Dinner			
Bedtime			
Snacks			

Friday

Time	Before	After	Notes
Breakfast			
Lunch			
Dinner			
Bedtime			
Snacks			

Saturday

Time	Before	After	Notes
Breakfast			
Lunch			
Dinner			
Bedtime			
Snacks			

Sunday

Time	Before	After	Notes
Breakfast			
Lunch			
Dinner			
Bedtime			
Snacks			

Notes

26.   Week:

Monday

Time	Before	After	Notes
Breakfast			
Lunch			
Dinner			
Bedtime			
Snacks			

Tuesday

Time	Before	After	Notes
Breakfast			
Lunch			
Dinner			
Bedtime			
Snacks			

Wednesday

Time	Before	After	Notes
Breakfast			
Lunch			
Dinner			
Bedtime			
Snacks			

Thursday

Time	Before	After	Notes
Breakfast			
Lunch			
Dinner			
Bedtime			
Snacks			

Friday

Time	Before	After	Notes
Breakfast			
Lunch			
Dinner			
Bedtime			
Snacks			

Saturday

Time	Before	After	Notes
Breakfast			
Lunch			
Dinner			
Bedtime			
Snacks			

Sunday

Time	Before	After	Notes
Breakfast			
Lunch			
Dinner			
Bedtime			
Snacks			

Notes

27.   Week:

Monday

Time	Before	After	Notes
Breakfast			
Lunch			
Dinner			
Bedtime			
Snacks			

Tuesday

Time	Before	After	Notes
Breakfast			
Lunch			
Dinner			
Bedtime			
Snacks			

Wednesday

Time	Before	After	Notes
Breakfast			
Lunch			
Dinner			
Bedtime			
Snacks			

Thursday

Time	Before	After	Notes
Breakfast			
Lunch			
Dinner			
Bedtime			
Snacks			

Friday

Time	Before	After	Notes
Breakfast			
Lunch			
Dinner			
Bedtime			
Snacks			

Saturday

Time	Before	After	Notes
Breakfast			
Lunch			
Dinner			
Bedtime			
Snacks			

Sunday

Time	Before	After	Notes
Breakfast			
Lunch			
Dinner			
Bedtime			
Snacks			

Notes

28.   Week:

Monday

Time	Before	After	Notes
Breakfast			
Lunch			
Dinner			
Bedtime			
Snacks			

Tuesday

Time	Before	After	Notes
Breakfast			
Lunch			
Dinner			
Bedtime			
Snacks			

Wednesday

Time	Before	After	Notes
Breakfast			
Lunch			
Dinner			
Bedtime			
Snacks			

Thursday

Time	Before	After	Notes
Breakfast			
Lunch			
Dinner			
Bedtime			
Snacks			

Friday

Time	Before	After	Notes
Breakfast			
Lunch			
Dinner			
Bedtime			
Snacks			

Saturday

Time	Before	After	Notes
Breakfast			
Lunch			
Dinner			
Bedtime			
Snacks			

Sunday

Time	Before	After	Notes
Breakfast			
Lunch			
Dinner			
Bedtime			
Snacks			

Notes

29.　Week:

Monday

Time	Before	After	Notes
Breakfast			
Lunch			
Dinner			
Bedtime			
Snacks			

Tuesday

Time	Before	After	Notes
Breakfast			
Lunch			
Dinner			
Bedtime			
Snacks			

Wednesday

Time	Before	After	Notes
Breakfast			
Lunch			
Dinner			
Bedtime			
Snacks			

Thursday

Time	Before	After	Notes
Breakfast			
Lunch			
Dinner			
Bedtime			
Snacks			

Friday

Time	Before	After	Notes
Breakfast			
Lunch			
Dinner			
Bedtime			
Snacks			

Saturday

Time	Before	After	Notes
Breakfast			
Lunch			
Dinner			
Bedtime			
Snacks			

Sunday

Time	Before	After	Notes
Breakfast			
Lunch			
Dinner			
Bedtime			
Snacks			

Notes

30. Week:

Monday

Time	Before	After	Notes
Breakfast			
Lunch			
Dinner			
Bedtime			
Snacks			

Tuesday

Time	Before	After	Notes
Breakfast			
Lunch			
Dinner			
Bedtime			
Snacks			

Wednesday

Time	Before	After	Notes
Breakfast			
Lunch			
Dinner			
Bedtime			
Snacks			

Thursday

Time	Before	After	Notes
Breakfast			
Lunch			
Dinner			
Bedtime			
Snacks			

Friday

Time	Before	After	Notes
Breakfast			
Lunch			
Dinner			
Bedtime			
Snacks			

Saturday

Time	Before	After	Notes
Breakfast			
Lunch			
Dinner			
Bedtime			
Snacks			

Sunday

Time	Before	After	Notes
Breakfast			
Lunch			
Dinner			
Bedtime			
Snacks			

Notes

31.   Week:

Monday

Time	Before	After	Notes
Breakfast			
Lunch			
Dinner			
Bedtime			
Snacks			

Tuesday

Time	Before	After	Notes
Breakfast			
Lunch			
Dinner			
Bedtime			
Snacks			

Wednesday

Time	Before	After	Notes
Breakfast			
Lunch			
Dinner			
Bedtime			
Snacks			

Thursday

Time	Before	After	Notes
Breakfast			
Lunch			
Dinner			
Bedtime			
Snacks			

Friday

Time	Before	After	Notes
Breakfast			
Lunch			
Dinner			
Bedtime			
Snacks			

Saturday

Time	Before	After	Notes
Breakfast			
Lunch			
Dinner			
Bedtime			
Snacks			

Sunday

Time	Before	After	Notes
Breakfast			
Lunch			
Dinner			
Bedtime			
Snacks			

Notes

32.   Week:

Monday

Time	Before	After	Notes
Breakfast			
Lunch			
Dinner			
Bedtime			
Snacks			

Tuesday

Time	Before	After	Notes
Breakfast			
Lunch			
Dinner			
Bedtime			
Snacks			

Wednesday

Time	Before	After	Notes
Breakfast			
Lunch			
Dinner			
Bedtime			
Snacks			

Thursday

Time	Before	After	Notes
Breakfast			
Lunch			
Dinner			
Bedtime			
Snacks			

Friday

Time	Before	After	Notes
Breakfast			
Lunch			
Dinner			
Bedtime			
Snacks			

Saturday

Time	Before	After	Notes
Breakfast			
Lunch			
Dinner			
Bedtime			
Snacks			

Sunday

Time	Before	After	Notes
Breakfast			
Lunch			
Dinner			
Bedtime			
Snacks			

Notes

33.   Week:

Monday

Time	Before	After	Notes
Breakfast			
Lunch			
Dinner			
Bedtime			
Snacks			

Tuesday

Time	Before	After	Notes
Breakfast			
Lunch			
Dinner			
Bedtime			
Snacks			

Wednesday

Time	Before	After	Notes
Breakfast			
Lunch			
Dinner			
Bedtime			
Snacks			

Thursday

Time	Before	After	Notes
Breakfast			
Lunch			
Dinner			
Bedtime			
Snacks			

Friday

Time	Before	After	Notes
Breakfast			
Lunch			
Dinner			
Bedtime			
Snacks			

Saturday

Time	Before	After	Notes
Breakfast			
Lunch			
Dinner			
Bedtime			
Snacks			

Sunday

Time	Before	After	Notes
Breakfast			
Lunch			
Dinner			
Bedtime			
Snacks			

Notes

34.   Week:

Monday

Time	Before	After	Notes
Breakfast			
Lunch			
Dinner			
Bedtime			
Snacks			

Tuesday

Time	Before	After	Notes
Breakfast			
Lunch			
Dinner			
Bedtime			
Snacks			

Wednesday

Time	Before	After	Notes
Breakfast			
Lunch			
Dinner			
Bedtime			
Snacks			

Thursday

Time	Before	After	Notes
Breakfast			
Lunch			
Dinner			
Bedtime			
Snacks			

Friday

Time	Before	After	Notes
Breakfast			
Lunch			
Dinner			
Bedtime			
Snacks			

Saturday

Time	Before	After	Notes
Breakfast			
Lunch			
Dinner			
Bedtime			
Snacks			

Sunday

Time	Before	After	Notes
Breakfast			
Lunch			
Dinner			
Bedtime			
Snacks			

Notes

35.   Week:

Monday

Time	Before	After	Notes
Breakfast			
Lunch			
Dinner			
Bedtime			
Snacks			

Tuesday

Time	Before	After	Notes
Breakfast			
Lunch			
Dinner			
Bedtime			
Snacks			

Wednesday

Time	Before	After	Notes
Breakfast			
Lunch			
Dinner			
Bedtime			
Snacks			

Thursday

Time	Before	After	Notes
Breakfast			
Lunch			
Dinner			
Bedtime			
Snacks			

Friday

Time	Before	After	Notes
Breakfast			
Lunch			
Dinner			
Bedtime			
Snacks			

Saturday

Time	Before	After	Notes
Breakfast			
Lunch			
Dinner			
Bedtime			
Snacks			

Sunday

Time	Before	After	Notes
Breakfast			
Lunch			
Dinner			
Bedtime			
Snacks			

Notes

36.   Week:

Monday

Time	Before	After	Notes
Breakfast			
Lunch			
Dinner			
Bedtime			
Snacks			

Tuesday

Time	Before	After	Notes
Breakfast			
Lunch			
Dinner			
Bedtime			
Snacks			

Wednesday

Time	Before	After	Notes
Breakfast			
Lunch			
Dinner			
Bedtime			
Snacks			

Thursday

Time	Before	After	Notes
Breakfast			
Lunch			
Dinner			
Bedtime			
Snacks			

Friday

Time	Before	After	Notes
Breakfast			
Lunch			
Dinner			
Bedtime			
Snacks			

Saturday

Time	Before	After	Notes
Breakfast			
Lunch			
Dinner			
Bedtime			
Snacks			

Sunday

Time	Before	After	Notes
Breakfast			
Lunch			
Dinner			
Bedtime			
Snacks			

Notes

37.   Week:

Monday

Time	Before	After	Notes
Breakfast			
Lunch			
Dinner			
Bedtime			
Snacks			

Tuesday

Time	Before	After	Notes
Breakfast			
Lunch			
Dinner			
Bedtime			
Snacks			

Wednesday

Time	Before	After	Notes
Breakfast			
Lunch			
Dinner			
Bedtime			
Snacks			

Thursday

Time	Before	After	Notes
Breakfast			
Lunch			
Dinner			
Bedtime			
Snacks			

Friday

Time	Before	After	Notes
Breakfast			
Lunch			
Dinner			
Bedtime			
Snacks			

Saturday

Time	Before	After	Notes
Breakfast			
Lunch			
Dinner			
Bedtime			
Snacks			

Sunday

Time	Before	After	Notes
Breakfast			
Lunch			
Dinner			
Bedtime			
Snacks			

Notes

38. Week:

Monday

Time	Before	After	Notes
Breakfast			
Lunch			
Dinner			
Bedtime			
Snacks			

Tuesday

Time	Before	After	Notes
Breakfast			
Lunch			
Dinner			
Bedtime			
Snacks			

Wednesday

Time	Before	After	Notes
Breakfast			
Lunch			
Dinner			
Bedtime			
Snacks			

Thursday

Time	Before	After	Notes
Breakfast			
Lunch			
Dinner			
Bedtime			
Snacks			

Friday

Time	Before	After	Notes
Breakfast			
Lunch			
Dinner			
Bedtime			
Snacks			

Saturday

Time	Before	After	Notes
Breakfast			
Lunch			
Dinner			
Bedtime			
Snacks			

Sunday

Time	Before	After	Notes
Breakfast			
Lunch			
Dinner			
Bedtime			
Snacks			

Notes

39.   Week:

Monday

Time	Before	After	Notes
Breakfast			
Lunch			
Dinner			
Bedtime			
Snacks			

Tuesday

Time	Before	After	Notes
Breakfast			
Lunch			
Dinner			
Bedtime			
Snacks			

Wednesday

Time	Before	After	Notes
Breakfast			
Lunch			
Dinner			
Bedtime			
Snacks			

Thursday

Time	Before	After	Notes
Breakfast			
Lunch			
Dinner			
Bedtime			
Snacks			

Friday

Time	Before	After	Notes
Breakfast			
Lunch			
Dinner			
Bedtime			
Snacks			

Saturday

Time	Before	After	Notes
Breakfast			
Lunch			
Dinner			
Bedtime			
Snacks			

Sunday

Time	Before	After	Notes
Breakfast			
Lunch			
Dinner			
Bedtime			
Snacks			

Notes

40. Week:

Monday

Time	Before	After	Notes
Breakfast			
Lunch			
Dinner			
Bedtime			
Snacks			

Tuesday

Time	Before	After	Notes
Breakfast			
Lunch			
Dinner			
Bedtime			
Snacks			

Wednesday

Time	Before	After	Notes
Breakfast			
Lunch			
Dinner			
Bedtime			
Snacks			

Thursday

Time	Before	After	Notes
Breakfast			
Lunch			
Dinner			
Bedtime			
Snacks			

Friday

Time	Before	After	Notes
Breakfast			
Lunch			
Dinner			
Bedtime			
Snacks			

Saturday

Time	Before	After	Notes
Breakfast			
Lunch			
Dinner			
Bedtime			
Snacks			

Sunday

Time	Before	After	Notes
Breakfast			
Lunch			
Dinner			
Bedtime			
Snacks			

Notes

41.   Week:

Monday

Time	Before	After	Notes
Breakfast			
Lunch			
Dinner			
Bedtime			
Snacks			

Tuesday

Time	Before	After	Notes
Breakfast			
Lunch			
Dinner			
Bedtime			
Snacks			

Wednesday

Time	Before	After	Notes
Breakfast			
Lunch			
Dinner			
Bedtime			
Snacks			

Thursday

Time	Before	After	Notes
Breakfast			
Lunch			
Dinner			
Bedtime			
Snacks			

Friday

Time	Before	After	Notes
Breakfast			
Lunch			
Dinner			
Bedtime			
Snacks			

Saturday

Time	Before	After	Notes
Breakfast			
Lunch			
Dinner			
Bedtime			
Snacks			

Sunday

Time	Before	After	Notes
Breakfast			
Lunch			
Dinner			
Bedtime			
Snacks			

Notes

42.   Week:

Monday

Time	Before	After	Notes
Breakfast			
Lunch			
Dinner			
Bedtime			
Snacks			

Tuesday

Time	Before	After	Notes
Breakfast			
Lunch			
Dinner			
Bedtime			
Snacks			

Wednesday

Time	Before	After	Notes
Breakfast			
Lunch			
Dinner			
Bedtime			
Snacks			

Thursday

Time	Before	After	Notes
Breakfast			
Lunch			
Dinner			
Bedtime			
Snacks			

Friday

Time	Before	After	Notes
Breakfast			
Lunch			
Dinner			
Bedtime			
Snacks			

Saturday

Time	Before	After	Notes
Breakfast			
Lunch			
Dinner			
Bedtime			
Snacks			

Sunday

Time	Before	After	Notes
Breakfast			
Lunch			
Dinner			
Bedtime			
Snacks			

Notes

43.   Week:

Monday

Time	Before	After	Notes
Breakfast			
Lunch			
Dinner			
Bedtime			
Snacks			

Tuesday

Time	Before	After	Notes
Breakfast			
Lunch			
Dinner			
Bedtime			
Snacks			

Wednesday

Time	Before	After	Notes
Breakfast			
Lunch			
Dinner			
Bedtime			
Snacks			

Thursday

Time	Before	After	Notes
Breakfast			
Lunch			
Dinner			
Bedtime			
Snacks			

Friday

Time	Before	After	Notes
Breakfast			
Lunch			
Dinner			
Bedtime			
Snacks			

Saturday

Time	Before	After	Notes
Breakfast			
Lunch			
Dinner			
Bedtime			
Snacks			

Sunday

Time	Before	After	Notes
Breakfast			
Lunch			
Dinner			
Bedtime			
Snacks			

Notes

44.   Week:

Monday

Time	Before	After	Notes
Breakfast			
Lunch			
Dinner			
Bedtime			
Snacks			

Tuesday

Time	Before	After	Notes
Breakfast			
Lunch			
Dinner			
Bedtime			
Snacks			

Wednesday

Time	Before	After	Notes
Breakfast			
Lunch			
Dinner			
Bedtime			
Snacks			

Thursday

Time	Before	After	Notes
Breakfast			
Lunch			
Dinner			
Bedtime			
Snacks			

Friday

Time	Before	After	Notes
Breakfast			
Lunch			
Dinner			
Bedtime			
Snacks			

Saturday

Time	Before	After	Notes
Breakfast			
Lunch			
Dinner			
Bedtime			
Snacks			

Sunday

Time	Before	After	Notes
Breakfast			
Lunch			
Dinner			
Bedtime			
Snacks			

Notes

45.   Week:

Monday

Time	Before	After	Notes
Breakfast			
Lunch			
Dinner			
Bedtime			
Snacks			

Tuesday

Time	Before	After	Notes
Breakfast			
Lunch			
Dinner			
Bedtime			
Snacks			

Wednesday

Time	Before	After	Notes
Breakfast			
Lunch			
Dinner			
Bedtime			
Snacks			

Thursday

Time	Before	After	Notes
Breakfast			
Lunch			
Dinner			
Bedtime			
Snacks			

Friday

Time	Before	After	Notes
Breakfast			
Lunch			
Dinner			
Bedtime			
Snacks			

Saturday

Time	Before	After	Notes
Breakfast			
Lunch			
Dinner			
Bedtime			
Snacks			

Sunday

Time	Before	After	Notes
Breakfast			
Lunch			
Dinner			
Bedtime			
Snacks			

Notes

46.   Week:

Monday

Time	Before	After	Notes
Breakfast			
Lunch			
Dinner			
Bedtime			
Snacks			

Tuesday

Time	Before	After	Notes
Breakfast			
Lunch			
Dinner			
Bedtime			
Snacks			

Wednesday

Time	Before	After	Notes
Breakfast			
Lunch			
Dinner			
Bedtime			
Snacks			

Thursday

Time	Before	After	Notes
Breakfast			
Lunch			
Dinner			
Bedtime			
Snacks			

Friday

Time	Before	After	Notes
Breakfast			
Lunch			
Dinner			
Bedtime			
Snacks			

Saturday

Time	Before	After	Notes
Breakfast			
Lunch			
Dinner			
Bedtime			
Snacks			

Sunday

Time	Before	After	Notes
Breakfast			
Lunch			
Dinner			
Bedtime			
Snacks			

Notes

47.   Week:

Monday

Time	Before	After	Notes
Breakfast			
Lunch			
Dinner			
Bedtime			
Snacks			

Tuesday

Time	Before	After	Notes
Breakfast			
Lunch			
Dinner			
Bedtime			
Snacks			

Wednesday

Time	Before	After	Notes
Breakfast			
Lunch			
Dinner			
Bedtime			
Snacks			

Thursday

Time	Before	After	Notes
Breakfast			
Lunch			
Dinner			
Bedtime			
Snacks			

Friday

Time	Before	After	Notes
Breakfast			
Lunch			
Dinner			
Bedtime			
Snacks			

Saturday

Time	Before	After	Notes
Breakfast			
Lunch			
Dinner			
Bedtime			
Snacks			

Sunday

Time	Before	After	Notes
Breakfast			
Lunch			
Dinner			
Bedtime			
Snacks			

Notes

48. Week:

Monday

Time	Before	After	Notes
Breakfast			
Lunch			
Dinner			
Bedtime			
Snacks			

Tuesday

Time	Before	After	Notes
Breakfast			
Lunch			
Dinner			
Bedtime			
Snacks			

Wednesday

Time	Before	After	Notes
Breakfast			
Lunch			
Dinner			
Bedtime			
Snacks			

Thursday

Time	Before	After	Notes
Breakfast			
Lunch			
Dinner			
Bedtime			
Snacks			

Friday

Time	Before	After	Notes
Breakfast			
Lunch			
Dinner			
Bedtime			
Snacks			

Saturday

Time	Before	After	Notes
Breakfast			
Lunch			
Dinner			
Bedtime			
Snacks			

Sunday

Time	Before	After	Notes
Breakfast			
Lunch			
Dinner			
Bedtime			
Snacks			

Notes

49.   Week:

Monday

Time	Before	After	Notes
Breakfast			
Lunch			
Dinner			
Bedtime			
Snacks			

Tuesday

Time	Before	After	Notes
Breakfast			
Lunch			
Dinner			
Bedtime			
Snacks			

Wednesday

Time	Before	After	Notes
Breakfast			
Lunch			
Dinner			
Bedtime			
Snacks			

Thursday

Time	Before	After	Notes
Breakfast			
Lunch			
Dinner			
Bedtime			
Snacks			

Friday

Time	Before	After	Notes
Breakfast			
Lunch			
Dinner			
Bedtime			
Snacks			

Saturday

Time	Before	After	Notes
Breakfast			
Lunch			
Dinner			
Bedtime			
Snacks			

Sunday

Time	Before	After	Notes
Breakfast			
Lunch			
Dinner			
Bedtime			
Snacks			

Notes

50.   Week:

Monday

Time	Before	After	Notes
Breakfast			
Lunch			
Dinner			
Bedtime			
Snacks			

Tuesday

Time	Before	After	Notes
Breakfast			
Lunch			
Dinner			
Bedtime			
Snacks			

Wednesday

Time	Before	After	Notes
Breakfast			
Lunch			
Dinner			
Bedtime			
Snacks			

Thursday

Time	Before	After	Notes
Breakfast			
Lunch			
Dinner			
Bedtime			
Snacks			

Friday

Time	Before	After	Notes
Breakfast			
Lunch			
Dinner			
Bedtime			
Snacks			

Saturday

Time	Before	After	Notes
Breakfast			
Lunch			
Dinner			
Bedtime			
Snacks			

Sunday

Time	Before	After	Notes
Breakfast			
Lunch			
Dinner			
Bedtime			
Snacks			

Notes

51.   Week:

Monday

Time	Before	After	Notes
Breakfast			
Lunch			
Dinner			
Bedtime			
Snacks			

Tuesday

Time	Before	After	Notes
Breakfast			
Lunch			
Dinner			
Bedtime			
Snacks			

Wednesday

Time	Before	After	Notes
Breakfast			
Lunch			
Dinner			
Bedtime			
Snacks			

Thursday

Time	Before	After	Notes
Breakfast			
Lunch			
Dinner			
Bedtime			
Snacks			

Friday

Time	Before	After	Notes
Breakfast			
Lunch			
Dinner			
Bedtime			
Snacks			

Saturday

Time	Before	After	Notes
Breakfast			
Lunch			
Dinner			
Bedtime			
Snacks			

Sunday

Time	Before	After	Notes
Breakfast			
Lunch			
Dinner			
Bedtime			
Snacks			

Notes

52. Week:

Monday

Time	Before	After	Notes
Breakfast			
Lunch			
Dinner			
Bedtime			
Snacks			

Tuesday

Time	Before	After	Notes
Breakfast			
Lunch			
Dinner			
Bedtime			
Snacks			

Wednesday

Time	Before	After	Notes
Breakfast			
Lunch			
Dinner			
Bedtime			
Snacks			

Thursday

Time	Before	After	Notes
Breakfast			
Lunch			
Dinner			
Bedtime			
Snacks			

Friday

Time	Before	After	Notes
Breakfast			
Lunch			
Dinner			
Bedtime			
Snacks			

Saturday

Time	Before	After	Notes
Breakfast			
Lunch			
Dinner			
Bedtime			
Snacks			

Sunday

Time	Before	After	Notes
Breakfast			
Lunch			
Dinner			
Bedtime			
Snacks			

Notes